HCG Diet Preparation:

Everything You Need To Know To Sucessfully Complete the HCG Diet & Lose Weight Fast!

Table of Contents

Introduction

I want to thank you and congratulate you for downloading the book, "*HCG Diet Preparation: Everything You Need To Know To Successfully Complete the HCG Diet and Lose Weight Fast!*"

This book contains proven steps and strategies on how to lose weight fast using the HCG diet plan.

This book will illustrate how the HCG treatment works and what you need to do to boost its effectiveness. As the HCG treatment cannot stand on its own in terms of weight loss, a strict diet plan is in place to ensure that you will get in that slim body that you have been dreaming of in a short amount of time. It may seem too good to be true but you just have to see for yourself how effective this weight loss program is.

To prepare you on your journey, this book is made so that you will know what to expect and what you should do in every phase of the HCG diet plan. You will get a feel of what the HCG diet is and why it is so effective. This book will explain why each phase in the diet plan is important and how you can benefit from the diet plan.

You need to understand that the HCG diet plan requires very strict adherence and this book will explain why and how you can cope with it. You will be given specific instructions on how you should plan your meals and the foods that you need to avoid.

This book will teach you how you can motivate yourself to be the healthier version of yourself. If becoming healthy is not enough to motivate you, this book will help you realize just how much you can gain when you reach your target weight.

This book should serve as your diet buddy all throughout your HCG diet plan journey. It has everything you need to know about the HCG treatment, the challenges, and how you can get past through those challenges.

This book will also serve as your guide as to how you can maintain your ideal weight once you are already there. There will be tips and life-changing realizations that you can learn by reading this book.

This book is better in hardback form because it comes with a weekly weight chart and daily journal located at the back of the book. You can use the weight chart to track your progress and note your HCG diet journey in the journal provided for you.

Thanks again for downloading this book. I hope you enjoy it!

Chapter 1: HCG Mindset Preparation

If you are one of those who have always been overweight their entire life or you simply want to lose the excess weight that you have gained over the past months, then here is a diet regimen that just might work for you. The HCG diet plan will allow you to lose the extra fat, and you will lose them fast. It may seem too far-fetched, but now, it is possible. By following a rigorous diet plan and taking the HCG supplement, you should be in your ideal weight in no time.

But first, let us go over the basics. HCG stands for human chorionic gonadotropin. It is the hormone produced during pregnancy that impedes a pregnant woman's feeling of hunger. By taking an HCG supplement, your body will respond the same way. You will not feel hungry right away and you will want smaller portions of food.

The hormone may also promote fat loss. Along with the HCG supplement, you will need to follow a very strict diet of 500 calories a day. This may seem too little as an average person needs at least 2000 calories daily. But the 500 calories a day is only during the first few days, at the time when you just have to burn the excess fats on your body. Once you are past this stage, you can gradually increase your calorie intake as described in the next chapters.

Before you jump into this diet plan, you will need to have a strong motivation why you have to lose the extra weight. This early on, you need to know that strictly adhering to the diet plan may prove to be tough. You will have to go through a serious change in your lifestyle that other people may find too difficult to follow. That is why you need to draw a clear picture of who you want to be before you start. And from there, you must use that to motivate yourself until you become that person.

Aside from the aesthetic benefits of following the diet plan, you also need to remember that being overweight is not healthy; not only physically, but mentally and emotionally as well. A lot of overweight people have to go through every day of their lives not liking the person they see on the mirror. If you are one of them, then it is time for you to take charge.

You need to know that it is possible to lose weight by following the diet, and maintain a healthy lifestyle. It is time to ditch the old mentality that you are just born fat and that there is nothing you can do about it. This is your body we are talking about and there is certainly something you can do.

To set your expectation, the road to achieving your ideal body may not be easy. This is the case for every diet plan there is. But the rewards of your hardships will be all worth it. As Sophocles once said, "There is no success without hardship." So to be that person you have illustrated on your mind, you have to work hard and follow the diet plan to a T.

Chapter 2: Why Do You Need To Be In This Diet Plan?

People who have used the HCG diet plan had made tremendous improvements in terms of the weighing scale. You can lose as much as one pound a day by sticking to the diet plan. Although the results may vary depending on the body mass and structure, you should see some improvement in as little as one week. You just have to see it for yourself and start the plan right away.

After weeks of being in the diet plan, you should see a better you that you never thought possible before. You can drastically change your future as you have gained a new-found confidence to face just about anything. Your confidence will stem from the fact that you have become a better version of yourself.

You will find more opportunities to be in any role you want; be it in a highly-competitive office, in the social scene, or having your own business. You will not have to catch your breath when going through a flight of stairs or drag yourself toward your destination because of the excess weight.

For some, there is a deep-seated motivation as to why they want to lose weight. You might be one of those who have always been bullied because you are overweight. You might have lost some career and life opportunities because of your weight. It is a known fact that obese people are being judged and discriminated in our society. You can change that by being healthier and leading a healthy lifestyle.

To be fully engaged in the HCG diet plan, you need to find your own motivation. If being healthier is not enough of a motivation, search deep within you so you will have the courage to stay in the diet plan no matter how hard it turns out to be. The first few weeks are the hardest and this is when it is easiest to quit. Find that motivation and hold on to it even after you have reached your goal. If you think getting to your desired weight is hard, maintaining it is even harder. But if you have hard-wired yourself that you want to be this person, then you should be able to get through it.

All throughout the process, you need to stay positive even if you do not lose at the same pace with other people. What is important is that you are seeing improvements, no matter how small they may be. It is not good to pit yourself with other people; this is your journey after all.

Every time you weigh yourself and see an improvement, you should be proud of yourself. You have worked so hard to be where you are and it should not be too long before you reach your desired weight. You need to understand that every person's body adapt and react in different ways. If you are strictly following the diet plan, then you are not doing anything wrong. It is just the way your body is adapting and reacting to the change in your lifestyle.

Chapter 3: The HCG Diet Plan

Before you start the HCG diet plan, you need to go through the loading phase first. The loading phase is where you eat everything you want until you feel very full. You should do this for a week before you start the treatment or until you have had your third injection. During this process, you will gain more weight but this should not cause alarm. You can lose all the additional weight, and more, during the entire process.

The reason behind the loading phase is because your body needs to have stored fat before you will be put in the 500 calorie diet. The reason that some people are unsuccessful in the HCG diet plan is because they went straight ahead for the 500 calorie diet. You need to understand that deposited fats only become available after the third injection. If you go into the 500 calorie diet without going through the loading phase first, then you will feel very weak as there is very little fat for your body to use.

The HCG diet plan requires you to adhere to a 500 calorie diet plan after the loading phase. Your diet consists of two meals per day. Your meal should have one protein, a piece of bread, one vegetable, and one fruit.

Your choices of protein include chicken breast, beef, veal, white fish, crab, lobster, or shrimp. The diet is strictly a no-fat diet so you should not eat any visible fat. Salmon, tuna, eel, herring, and pickled or dried fish are not allowed.

Your bread should be a piece of Melba toast or one breadstick.

For the vegetables, you can have beet greens, spinach, green salad, chard, celery, chicory, tomatoes, onions, fennel, cucumbers, red radish, cabbage, or asparagus.

As for the fruit, you have a choice between an apple, an orange, a few pieces of strawberries, or a half slice of a grapefruit.

You can have as much water as you want. You can also have tea or black coffee but milk should be limited to 1 tablespoon a day. Sugar substitutes are allowed. However, oil, butter, and sugar are not. The only methods allowed in cooking your food are by broiling or grilling them. Definitely no frying allowed.

The key here is that you are eating only because you are hungry. You need to think of the people in the old days when they only eat when they feel like they are hungry. And before they do, they need to look for their food or they eat as they go on their way. This is what you are trying to teach your body -- to eat only when you have to. You should be able to resist eating everything on sight. In the old days, food is not always readily available. People's methods of preparing food are also limited because they do not have the equipment or resources to prepare their food in other ways. It's hard but you can do it – and it will be so worth it. You will see, soon enough. Just keep this in mind when faced with very little choices in food.

Chapter 4: Tracking Your Weekly Progress

During the first few weeks of the HCG diet plan, it is important to track your weekly progress. You can easily feel discouraged if your body does not show any sign of improvement. However, not until you step into a weighing scale will you know that there is actually an improvement. The physical improvements will not be visible right away. You have to stay patient and track your weekly progress so you will stay motivated. Aside from the motivations you have outlined in Chapters 1 and 2, your weekly progress should be a form of motivation in itself.

You can use the weight chart at the end of this book to track your weekly progress. Writing down your progress will give you a better feel of how you are doing. You can actually compare your data week after week and use those improvements to further your journey.

You should also take progress pictures. Start with right before you start the HCG diet plan until you reach your target weight. A visual reminder of how you were before and where you are right now should be a motivating factor for you to keep on pushing.

You will also need to buy a weighing scale and use it weekly so you will see how you tip the scale. Your weighing scale should be your diet buddy that can give you unbiased and accurate answers to whether you are losing weight or not. A weighing scale is essential in tracking your progress. Without a weighing scale, you will just have to guess how you are doing.

Aside from the motivating factors provided by tracking your progress, you will also know whether the plan is working for you. You may feel skeptical at first, especially when there are no visible improvements. But if you have a written and photographic evidence of how you are doing, then you will know every inch of improvement that you are going through.

You can even use your progress as proof so you can help other people who also want to lose weight. Some people need hard evidence before they believe anything to be true, and this is not a bad thing at all. You also need to practice the same thing so you will not get trapped into a diet plan that does not work for you.

Our bodies work in different ways. Another person's body may respond positively to a specific diet plan while others do not. While some diet plans are not really designed to work, some may offer great results. You should totally skip the diet plans that do not work. The trick is finding the plan that actually works and ensuring that it will work on you. The only way to know for sure is by tracking your progress. You should also keep tabs of what you can do more so you can get to your desired weight in the least amount of time without sacrificing your health.

Chapter 5: Getting Through the HCG Diet

As with any other diet plan, there are the challenging parts. These are the times when you feel that you are doing so much but producing very little results. But most people quit right after they started.

For one, the early days are usually the hardest part. This is when you have to make changes and changes do come very hard. And once you feel that challenge, you may tend to quit right away thinking that you have not invested that much anyway, so it's okay to give up.

The thing is, it is not okay. It is not okay to live throughout your life feeling defeated. To think that there is nothing you can do is unacceptable. You have to dig deep and decide that you want to change your life. You can change your destiny by sticking to what you really want instead of settling to what is comfortable for you.

As with the HCG diet plan, the hardest part is sticking to a strict calorie limit. Food is readily available for you and your instinct is to grab that food and have a bite. If you intend to go through the HCG diet plan, the food mentality of grab and go will not work. You have to follow the diet described in Chapter 3 to achieve the results that you want. You should not worry about feeling hungry as the HCG hormone will help you to not feel the hunger.

For the HCG diet plan to work, you need to strictly follow all the procedures. If necessary, you may need to admit yourself in the clinic where your shots will be administered. This is to ensure that you are given the shots you need and that your food is prepared the way it should be and in the right amount. You do not have to be confined in the hospital all day. You are allowed to leave and stroll around as long as you do not consume food while you are out of the hospital. Nevertheless, it is also perfectly fine to be an outpatient, given that you have the strength and motivation to stick to the plan despite all the food around you.

You do not have to be in the 500 calorie diet all throughout. After finishing the diet plan, you can resume to regular eating as long as you restrict your intake of starch and sugar.

During the course of your treatment with HCG, you will not be required to work out because the low calorie diet will have to use the stored fats in your body for energy. However, after the treatment, you can work out to reduce the appearance of sagging skin. You can start to build muscles after you have achieved your ideal weight. Working out is also a good way to burn up calories since you would have resumed to regular eating by then. This will also aid in maintaining your weight so you will not feel like a failure once your weight goes up again.

After the HCG treatment, it is up to you to take care of yourself. And taking of yourself includes watching what you eat and working out.

Chapter 6: The HCG Diet Learning Curve

The HCG Diet Learning Curve consists of four phases. You must follow each phase religiously so you will have success with the HCG diet plan.

The first phase is the loading phase. The loading phase will encourage you to consume high calorie foods so you can build up stored fats. For most people, this is the most enjoyable part as they get to eat everything they want. However, some people are very skeptical about the loading phase that they tend to skip it totally. By doing so, they are risking themselves of having to deal with loss of strength at the start of the diet plan because they have not prepared their bodies for the low calorie diet. It is important to note that the loading phase is not simply a way to eat to your heart's delight. The rationale behind it lies in the fact that when you turn into the low calorie diet, your body must have stored fats that it can burn for energy.

The second phase is the most challenging phase and it can last from 23 to a maximum of 40 days. It is in this phase that the 500 calorie diet is introduced. Although the HCG hormone reduces a person's appetite for food, some may find it hard to resist eating even when they are not really hungry. Aside from the eating habits that you have developed, your social setting can also directly impact the success of the diet plan. Social setting includes the eating habits of the people you are always with, the availability of the food around you, and other stress-related eating habits. Understanding the triggers of unplanned eating will help you find ways to manage them. For example, if you eat every time your workmates are eating, then you may need pass on the next meal and always remind yourself that you should not eat outside your diet plan.

The third phase is the stabilization phase. In this phase, you will no longer be given the HCG treatment but you will still need to watch your weight. It may be necessary to take your daily weight to see if your body is holding up to your ideal weight. If you see increases in your weight, you may need to get in touch with your doctor so he can give you further guidelines as to how you can maintain your weight.

The fourth, and final, phase is the maintenance phase. This phase is extremely important as it will be all up to you how you can keep your weight. You need to be conscious about not going back to your old eating habits that caused your excess weight. It is in this phase that the HCG diet plan will teach you how you can maintain your weight for good. From this point on, you will need to have a balanced diet and a healthier lifestyle. This is also the phase that you can have a less restrictive diet. You can also start to work out during this phase so you can tone your body and improve it further more.

To get past all these phases, you will need to strictly adhere to the diet plan while monitoring your progress. A doctor's guidance all throughout the four phases may be beneficial to ensuring that you are doing things the right way. But this is not a requirement. Some people achieved success by simply following the protocols of the diet plan. You just need to do what works best for you and with what you are more comfortable with. If in case you feel that something is off, consult with a doctor immediately.

You will also need to be patient with yourself if the improvements of the diet plan do not translate right away to your appearance. Your body may be adjusting in a different manner; that is why your progress is not visible. By continuously adhering to the program, you should see physical improvements within weeks. You should not give up on yourself right away.

The HCG diet plan may work best by under the close supervision of a medical practitioner. There may be some side effects to this diet plan but these side effects can be managed with the help of a doctor who understands the process.

Your body will also undergo a learning curve as it get used to the 500 calorie diet. You have been forewarned in the earlier chapters of this book that the challenge is at its greatest when your body is starting to adjust to the new diet plan. You may feel the urge to eat even when you are not hungry. Little by little, you will need to distinguish real hunger from hunger caused by the habit you were used to. You should not worry about this as this may become easier for you with the aid of the HCG treatment and as your body tries to adjust to the new diet plan. The HCG treatment should minimize hunger pains and will reduce the feelings of hunger. Your body's learning curve will help you to adapt to the rigorous diet plan and you will feel more comfortable as you go along.

Chapter 7: Post-HCG Diet Plan

After you have achieved your ideal weight, one of the challenges of being in the post HCG diet plan is knowing how to move forward. After the HCG diet plan, you will be allowed to have regular portions of food. You should not be overly excited about this and begin eating everything that you want. You should remember that the reason you were overweight before is because of your poor eating habits. You should not over-indulge thinking that your body will not go back to where it was before. It is an ever-looming possibility especially if you do not take good measures to maintain your weight.

After the HCG diet plan, you should be more conscious with what you eat. You should follow a low-fat diet and limit your consumption of starchy foods and sugar. You can also start to work out so you can have a more toned and healthy body. One of the main reasons that your body stores up fat is that the sugars you consume are not converted into energy. By working out, you are enabling your body to use up calories and any excess fat so they do not get stored in your body which could eventually cause obesity.

Being overweight should be a thing in the past for you once you reach this stage. You should be more motivated to keep your body because you worked hard for it and you deserve it. Do not let all your hard work go to waste by neglecting your body and forgetting what the HCG diet plan has taught you.

Having a healthy body is a product of a healthy lifestyle. Everything that you put in your mouth will be reflected in your figure and in the weighing scale so you need to choose well and choose right. You should not consume foods that are not needed by your body. Eat right and eat when you have to. You should know by now how you can interpret your body's needs. There is no need to eat when you are not hungry. You need to remove the habit of binge eating as it adds to much of your weight.

You should eat to nourish your body. Eating should not be a means to cure your boredom or to manage your emotions. You need to find other ways to pass the time.

You can start to pick up a hobby and become busy so you can take your mind off from eating unnecessarily. You may also need to find other ways to manage your stress and emotions. Being an emotional eater is not healthy as you tend to consume more food to make yourself feel better. The reality here is that overeating will not take all your problems away. And overeating may impose another problem for you.

Ultimately, having a healthy body solves a myriad of things for you. You get to enjoy the tangible benefits of having a great figure. Aside from that, you get to love yourself more and have the feeling that you are in charge. You are healthy physically, mentally, and emotionally.

Your Weight Loss Chart And Journal

Instructions in using the weight loss chart

Materials:

For the weight loss chart, you will need the chart, a weighing scale, a pen, and lots of motivation and perseverance.

Procedures:

1. Fill in the month's column. Write what month of the year it is so you will know when you started and you can have a record of your monthly progress.

2. Under the Week Column, you should write the week number that you are currently in. You should record your week number at the end of every week. Your first entry should be Week 0. Your next entry will be Week 1 and that is 7 days after you recorded your initial weight.

3. On the Weight Column, you should write the weight registered on your weighing scale at the end of every week. Your first entry should be your weight prior to starting the diet plan. The next entry will be your weight at the end of the following weeks.

4. The Goal Weight Column should contain your target weight at the end of every week. Do not create goals that are too high or too low. You need the right amount of motivation to keep you afloat. Setting a goal that is too high may dampen your spirit especially when you are not meeting them week after week. But setting a goal that is too low may also set the wrong expectations. When setting your goal, you must be realistic.

5. Under the Goal Met? Column, you just need to write if your weight at the end of the week matches you goal weight. This is just a Yes and No Column.

6. Under the Notes, you will need to write your observations every week and deviations from the diet plan, if any. You can also note the difference in your weight and goal weight to see how far you are from where you want to

be in a weekly basis. You can also write your progress as compared with the previous week under the Notes Column.

Instructions in using the journal

Your journal should keep a record of everything that is related to your HCG diet plan. You can write the schedules of your injections in your journal. You can also write down your meal plans and keep a record of all the food you eat, no matter how small you think they are. You can use your journal to keep track of your calorie intake.

Everything should be recorded in your journal so once it is time to step on the weighing scale, you will know exactly why you are in that weight. You should write a line every day no matter how irrelevant you think it may be. At the end of the week, that irrelevant information may tell you a lot. If the information is related to your HCG diet plan, write it.

Weight Loss Chart				
Month:				
Week	Weight	Goal Weight	Goal Met? Yes/No	Notes

Weight Loss Chart				
Month:				
Week	Weight	Goal Weight	Goal Met? Yes/No	Notes

Your HCG Diet Plan Journal

_____

_____

_____

_____

_____

_____

_____

_____

_____

_____

_____

_____

_____

_____

_____

_____

_____

_____

_____

_____

_____

_____

Your HCG Diet Plan Journal

_____

_____

_____

_____

_____

_____

_____

_____

_____

_____

_____

_____

_____

_____

_____

_____

_____

_____

_____

_____

_____

_____

_____

_____

Your HCG Diet Plan Journal

_____

_____

_____

_____

_____

_____

_____

_____

_____

_____

_____

_____

_____

_____

_____

_____

_____

_____

_____

_____

Your HCG Diet Plan Journal

_____

_____

_____

_____

_____

_____

_____

_____

_____

_____

_____

_____

_____

_____

_____

_____

_____

_____

_____

_____

_____

Your HCG Diet Plan Journal

Conclusion

Thank you again for downloading this book!

I hope this book was able to help you to understand the HCG diet plan and prepare you for your journey. The diet plan may be a tough process that you will have to go through but the intrinsic rewards are endless. Every time you feel that you have to give up, just imagine the the person you will be after the diet plan. That is the person you are giving up.

The next step is to start with the process of the diet plan by following the procedures illustrated in this book. You will need to strictly follow all the phases as each of them are sensible and proven to aid in your weight loss.

You should have the confidence to start with the HCG diet plan as you are now well-equipped with all the knowledge and motivation necessary to start the plan. If in any stage of the program you feel like doubting yourself, feel free to pick this book up again and read it so you can have a reminder why you are doing what you are doing. You should have this book on your entire journey so you will not have a chance to doubt whether what you are doing is beneficial for you.

Being overweight is not healthy. And by following the HCG diet plan, you are on your way to a healthier you and you can be there fast.

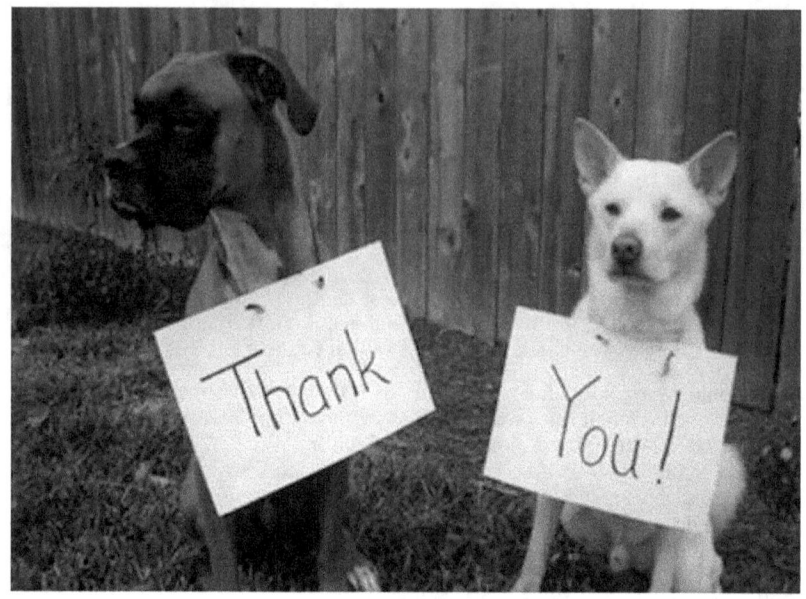

Finally, if you enjoyed this book, then I'd like to ask you for a favor, would you be kind enough to leave a review for this book on Amazon? It'd be greatly appreciated!

Click here to leave a review for this book on Amazon!

Thank you and good luck!